EATING HEALTHY FOR LIFE

A practical approach especially for busy people, overweight, skinny, emotional binge eater, and even alcoholic...

Aeshire Charles & Ishita Lohani

CHAPTERS:

INTRODUCTION

Disclaimer: This book might be too awesome for your soul. It has unforeseen practical tips and is customized for the many types of people in this world.

You're probably having a fabulous lifestyle with all the luxuries of the world. 20-30 somethings are surviving their competitive lives by the age- old formulae of working their asses off on weekdays and binge drinking on weekends completing it by sleeping the whole Sunday. Those who have had their share of these days are struggling hard to live a healthier life with a nice schedule and everything.

But it is sure hard, isn't it?

The essence of healthy living lies in one thing- HEALTHY EATING. It is again not easy to eat healthy all along. Although it is very important that we realize the importance of eating healthy.

This book is not simply written to make you eat healthier, it is carefully 'crafted' to explain to you how you can 'easily' start eating healthier and follow it for the rest of your life without putting in it any extra effort. Pretty smooth right?

How does this book help you? From our experiences the biggest challenges for us to help our clients live a healthy life was to explain to them the real idea of eating healthy. So the chapter of this book would make you realize the true meaning of eating healthy, the definitions and the processes involved are the same.

Then we come to the REAL part of the book. The reason we thought of writing this book in the first place was because people try hard to do the 'ideal' thing. The ideal is unreal. It is the deviation from reality. All of the books would be about the practical things you can do to eat the best things for yourself. It will also take care of the fact that people are different. So if you are busy, or you are fat, or you are so thin that people call you undernourished, or you have anger issues which need binge eating rounds to calm your insides, OR if you hate the idea of healthy eating. This book has something for everyone in its stores.

CHAPTERS YOU NEED TO FOLLOW TO EAT HEALTHY FOR A LONGER LIFE

1.   UNDERSTANDING HEALTHY EATING

A healthy diet, as the phrase itself suggests, is eating nutritious or healthy food, in short. Fair enough, but what does it actually mean?

You, the reader, of this book, are probably a grown ass man in his late 30's, or a teenage girl trying to stay in her best figure, or an overweight college guy wanting some appreciation and not just shunning. But healthy eating is not just for these people. As food experts, we wanna make this clear to you that eating healthy food benefits not just the body, but the future generations that your bloodline is gonna be responsible for.

For healthy eating, we need to focus on not just food, but the type of food and the nutrition value it has. In a single item of food, we have to look at ingredients such as a number of proteins, carbohydrates, sugar, fat, salts... you get the point. Every person on this planet has a different nutritional requirement just as he/she has a unique fingerprint (granted the nutritional needs may vary slightly to heavily considering the physique of the person involved).

Let's start talking technically here. We're gonna stick to a very simplified jargon of the food nutritionists, so do not worry.

Daily amounts that an average human being is recommended so that he/she can achieve a balanced and a healthy diet to maintain rather than gain or lose weight is called Reference Intake (RI). The energy reference intake, which is the average daily intake of energy needed for an average male, is 2500 kilocalories (kcal) while it is 2000 kcal for an average female. For our non-science readers, we would like to explain that 1 calorie roughly equals the energy required to lift 500 grams of water vertically by 1 meter. If you're on your calculator figuring out daily how much water an average human needs to lift vertically, then don't. That's not relevant. Our actual point is that energy requirements for an average male and female differ by 25 percent. Below is a table of the average reference intakes of humans.

	Men	Women
Energy (kcal)	2500	2000
Protein (g)	55	50
Carbohydrates (g)	300	260
Sugar (g)	120	90
Fat (g)	95	70
Saturates (g)	30	20
Salt (g)	6	6

A normal businessman who's reading this book is gonna be so pissed at us for using kcal as the reference of measurement instead of the actual portion size. So, we'll try to explain using your actual body part.

Foods which contain carbohydrates like potato, pasta, cereal, rice, etc should have a rough serving size of YOUR fist (don't loosen that fist just because you love that pasta). Foods containing protein such as poultry, meat or fish should have a portion size of your hand's palm. Again, we would like to point out that these sizes are rough estimates of the actual reference intakes.

Popcorn, chips or other savouries should have a serving size of a pair formed by your cupped hands. Bakes such as brownies and cakes or flapjacks must be served at a size of your two fingers (Yep! Take that, diabetes!).

Finally, butter and other spreads should have a portion size of your thumb's tip.

It's best that the hand used in the above references belong to the person who's gonna be served the meal.

Since we have successfully dealt with the science of the required nutrients, we can now transition to the actual meals an average person takes in a day.

Breakfast. The word breakfast literally breaks down to two meager words in the English language, "break" and "fast". A breakfast is supposed to, or often, is needed to jump-start your metabolic activities after a good night sleep or a hard night of partying and the following hangover. One should include a protein diet such as salmon, eggs, and other dairy products to get the blood sugar rolling. Always remember that you should never skip this important part of your meal as it makes up the ground for the other foods that you're gonna eat eventually during the day.

Mid-Morning. Though this snack party is enjoyed by a very small percentage of people on this planet, it still is a necessary and a crucial meal required in the overall eating regimen. This meal is usually to evenly spread the nutrition intake into broken small meals so that the sugar in the blood is evenly distributed and has enough time to be processed by the body and not forced. Peanut butter topped morning biscuits or bananas are good options for a mid-morning meal and can be accompanied by some veggie sticks.

Lunch. The lunch is one of the most important meals of the day. One should fill his/her lunch with proteins and sugary carbohydrates. Lunch needs to provide the required energy or else you're gonna get sloppy the whole afternoon. A friendly advice would be to choose sugary carbohydrates to successfully raise the sugar in the bloodstream. Whole grain fiber foods are recommended, such as salmon or chicken topped sandwiches, dressed with salad to help the liquid intake as well.

Mid-Afternoon. This contains the sweet afternoon munchies which satisfy the need for the energy with some fruit. Apple rings (dried), walnuts and almonds are the perfect food for this meal. Dried fruits contain nearly four times as much sugar as their fresh counterparts have. Also, low-calorie fruits such as tomatoes, cherries, apples can be consulted instead of that biscuit box if one fancies something crunchy and sweet.

Dinner. This is the most important meal of the whole day. This meal follows a long night rest where the body suspends its functions and hibernates for hours. One should not abandon carbohydrates in dinner as they're low fat and help the body in repair and rejuvenation after a whole night of decomposition and processing. A healthy, carbohydrate-rich dinner maintains the skin glowing and hair healthy. One can have fish, beans or meat with a plate full of various salads and veggies.

2. MUCH NEEDED MYTH BUSTING

"Do not drink water after eating cucumber, you'll get cholera"...

"Spicy foods in the dinner are not good for health"...
Myth busting is a tedious task since people usually come up with bizarre myths and rumors of healthy eating lifestyle that even food experts think twice to talk about. But since we're here and discussed the prerequisites of healthy eating in the last chapter, we might as well debunk some fake myths the public have regarding nutrition.

- **"One needs to keep a count on calories to lose weight".**
Okay. First of all, 50 calories of brownies and soda are not equivalent to 50 calories of broccoli or rice. Losing weight is a meticulous yet easy task that involves providing the body with required vitamins and minerals, but abandoning the fat and carbohydrates that may chip in the body fat. To lose weight, one has to schedule his/her meals with caution as per the above statement. The number of calories does not matter. What matters is the source of those calories, that is the food item that you're consuming. The obsession with calorie counting will get you nowhere.

- **"Having a meal after 6 pm causes weight gain".**
This myth is as untrue as the previous one just because it works around the premise of when to eat, and not what to eat. The time of eating is usually never a problem unless your

meals are 12 hours apart. The actual problem arises when people eat so late that they're already starving and they end up overeating. Overeating causes weight gain. That's no myth. If you consume more than required calories at 4pm too, you're gonna gain weight.

- **"A low carbohydrate or even a no carbohydrate diet is good for health".**

This statement is just plain stupid. Carbohydrates, just as fat, sugar, minerals, vitamins, etc. are needed by the body for its proper functioning. Even the brain needs carbohydrates to function properly. It's the refined carbohydrates (such as cookies, white bread, etc.) that can be curfewed or abandoned. But sources of healthy carbohydrates, for instance, vegetables, whole grains, fruits are particularly needed by every human being.

- **"Nutritional value of frozen vegetables and fruits is less than the fresh ones".**

When vegetables and fruits are picked, they are systematically flash-frozen so that majority of the nutrients are locked inside them. Fresh fruits are obviously preferred and advised over frozen foods but if someone's in a rush or if it's not the season or if he/she can't buy the fresh items because of some reason, their frozen counterparts can get the job done.

- **"Eating small and frequent meals throughout the day controls the metabolism better than having larger and fewer meals".**

This is probably the most common myth that's associated with healthy eating. Every time we eat something, our metabolism kick-starts as the body starts processing what we have eaten. That means that small and frequent meals would gear up our metabolism more often and burn some calories every time. But the meals are small so the calorie intake doesn't really add up too much. On the other hand, frequent meals cause dieters to keep the digestive gears grinding and they don't overeat if they finally sit down to have a bite. But, for other consumers, discipline and control are an ability they lose every time they eat. So, it really comes down to the person and he/she is the one who chooses the eating pattern.

- **"Microwave oven takes out the nutritional value".**

This myth is just an ignorant and a misguided comment. First of all, we need to understand what microwave ovens do. Microwaves are electromagnetic radiation, that is invisible light (like your TV remote uses) and these ovens emit these radiations throughout and evenly to produce heat. Now, the loss of nutrients depends on how long and how vigorously the food item is being heated, rather than where it is heated. The more time you heat the food item, the more it loses nutrients. Since microwaving actually speeds up the heating process, it actually preserves the nutritional value of the food.

- **"Calories that are consumed at night time damage more than those taken in the daytime".**

What? Calories are and will be calories at any time of the day. What matters is a number of calories that a person takes. Also, calories do not damage the human body, it's overeating or over-consumption of calories that adds up to body fat.

- **"Eggs are responsible for heart diseases".**

Eggs do have yolk in them which has a considerable amount of cholesterol in it - roughly 200 mg in a large egg. And yes, the fatty stuff that clogs up our arteries and causes heart attacks is famously called cholesterol. But connecting these two sentences is misguided. For one, the cholesterol that's present in our food items such as eggs, etc., isn't really responsible for the clogging up of heart arteries. This cholesterol is compensated by the body automatically as it commands itself to manufacture less cholesterol. So what causes heart attacks, you ask... Well, it's the cholesterol that's found in trans fats and saturated fats. They have a heavy impact on the blood cholesterol levels. That being said, the cholesterol intake of an average human being should be limited to 300 milligrams daily.

- **"Obesity is caused by the inability of the body to process dairy or wheat".**

This myth just collapsed in on itself. If the body cannot process dairy (milk and stuff), then the loss of nutrients and non-absorption of calories will cause the body to lose weight and not gain. The problem associated with this myth is "food allergy". And we still don't have any scientific or experimental evidence that food allergies cause weight gain.

3.   QUITTING YOUR IDEAL NOTIONS

There are many people who start with healthy eating with expectations that never get fulfilled. The reason is simple, they have unreal bookish expectations from their health goals. Well, one might think that this is not common but in reality, we being nutrition experts have seen many many people all over the years who come disappointed because they had wrong notions of staying fit. They had schedules so strict that everything started piling up and then what comes is a disappointment.

So many of the people who feel disappointed by themselves for not doing the planned thing, also start feeling bad by themselves and this, combined with the societal pressure, leads them into calling themselves a failure. When this happens, they usually lose inhibitions and care and eat whatever comes in their way. Either this happens or anorexia! Both are extremely harmful situations and have the potential to cause deadly problems in future. So our job here is to prevent that from happening. How do we do that? By explaining people that being maniacs about things in life is not a great idea. The idea of a good health stands precisely so that you can enjoy it. Even if you have not taken care of your health previously, then it does not mean you will overexert yourself and set unreal goals and deadlines.

Now we believe you got our point, so let us come to the main point. How do you form a plan for yourself which is practical, not ideal? It becomes a bit of a deal because this is not a process where you can just read about your future schedule somewhere and start following it. You have to sit, and by trial and error make it for yourself. We are here telling you the basics and we will also tell you how you should go on making a proper schedule for yourself where you can eat healthily and live healthily!

- Well, first of all, it is important that you know what ideally is good for the various kinds of people around. For that you need to know two things, number 1 is what are the various kinds of people around in terms of nutrition or type of their bodies and the other recommended dietary allowances also called as RDA. Coming to the first thing, there are actually 3 types of body types. One is an endomorph, then the ectomorph and one is a mesomorph. The endomorph is the one which has a comparatively slower metabolism and carries more fat. Ectomorphs are usually skinny people who have fiery metabolisms and digest anything you provide them. The mesomorphs as you can decipher fall somewhere in the between. They are the ones with the appropriate amount of fat naturally and some muscle which makes them look good and healthy. This is because they neither have a low or a fiery metabolism. It is important to know this because all three of them significantly differ in their nutritional requirements.

- **Here is how you should go about this:** Ectomorphs should be consuming more amount of carbohydrates, appropriate amounts of proteins and lesser fats. This less fat thing might sound weird but carbohydrates make the real difference which actually has been explained in good detail in the overweight and underweight sections! For the mesomorphs, literally everything in equal proportions rocks. Their bodies are doing great and they just need to carry on. Coming to endomorphs, some of the most worried people on earth. Yes! It is sad but not all hope is lost, your body has a lot of energy which needs to be spent, so basically if the endomorphs cut on their carb intake and increase the protein and fat intake, they would get in shape easily.

For Ectomorph Men

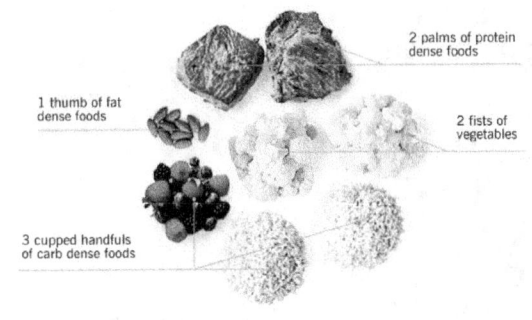

2 palms of protein dense foods

1 thumb of fat dense foods

2 fists of vegetables

3 cupped handfuls of carb dense foods

Image source: Precision Nutrition

For Ectomorph Women

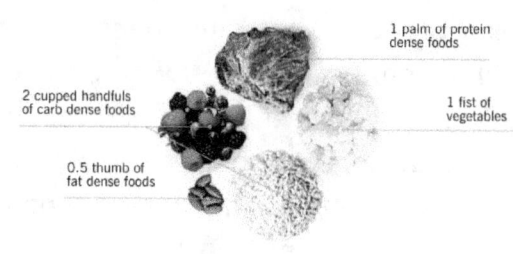

1 palm of protein dense foods

2 cupped handfuls of carb dense foods

1 fist of vegetables

0.5 thumb of fat dense foods

Image source: Precision Nutrition

For Mesomorph Men

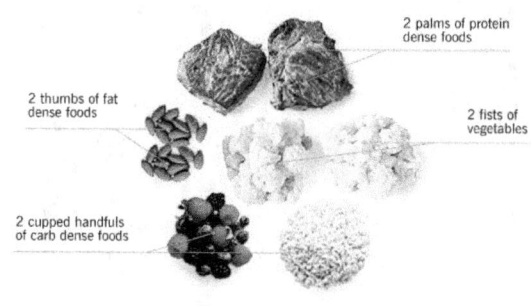

2 palms of protein dense foods

2 thumbs of fat dense foods

2 fists of vegetables

2 cupped handfuls of carb dense foods

Image source: Precision Nutrition

For Mesomorph Women

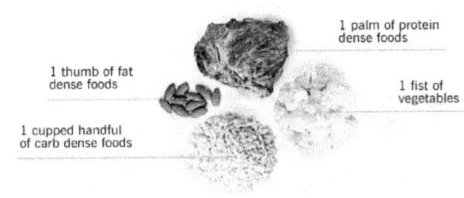

1 thumb of fat
dense foods

1 palm of protein
dense foods

1 fist of
vegetables

1 cupped handful
of carb dense foods

Image source: Precision Nutrition

For Endomorph Men

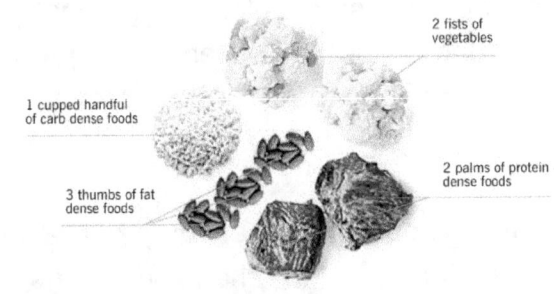

2 fists of
vegetables

1 cupped handful
of carb dense foods

2 palms of protein
dense foods

3 thumbs of fat
dense foods

Image source: Precision Nutrition

For Endomorph Women

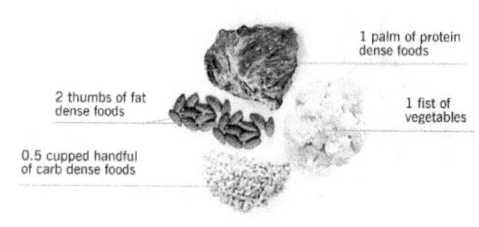

2 thumbs of fat
dense foods

0.5 cupped handful
of carb dense foods

1 palm of protein
dense foods

1 fist of
vegetables

Image source: Precision Nutrition

- So, the second thing we had to keep in our minds was the recommended dietary allowance or the RDA is actually average intake of nutrients for a day. So one before opting for healthy eating should have some idea about what are the requirements of our body. Not that we are saying if it is 10g then you cannot consume 9.5g, but you should know that 10g is good for you.

- How do you go about eating healthy practically? Well, we have taken the first step in changing things in this scenario. We know what is out body type and how much of what one should consume. So now you need to understand that you might now exactly fit in one body type, or you might fall between mesomorph and ectomorph, this is something you can easily tell. But then you have to tailor the diet for yourself. First of all, make a list of all things you love to eat. Then make a list of all the things you don't like to eat. Make a list of the healthy things like vegetables and milk and fruits. After this you make a meal plan you think you will be able to follow!

- **Here is an 8-week diet plan which anyone of you can look for as an example!**

MONTH 1 :

days	8:00 am breakfast	11:30 am	2:00 pm	AFTER GYM	8:00 pm
1	2 eggs omelette. Full glass of milk. 2 Bread Pieces. 2 almonds and 2 walnuts	Sprout Salad Green Tea	Dry chickpea salad; boiled cumin and garlic potatoes	Any fruit	Small salad, egg curry.
2	Chicken Sandwich (No mayo or fatty dressings, use as many vegetables as	Carrot Sticks with Dip: ½ cup carrot	Tuna- Cucumber Wrap 5 cucumber sticks ¼ cup low-	Any fruit	Vegetable soupy oats

	you can) Orange Juice.	sticks 2 Tbsp hummus Green Tea	fat vanilla yogurt		
3	Blueberry pancakes and a tall glass of cold mocha latte.	1 large orange 2 graham crackers Green Tea	Oven sweet potato fries with mint and coriander sauce.	Any fruit	One Pan Spaghetti (includes ground beef and tomato sauce)
4	Muesli or any cereal of choice with milk, a small salad.	Sprout salad Green Tea	Cottage Cheese in onion tomato gravy.	Any fruit	Vegetable and soybean Thukpa
5	Vegetable Sandwich plus a glass of buttermilk	Carrot Sticks with Dip: ½	Small salad, egg curry, bread 2 pieces.	Any fruit	Soupy Vegetable Oats

		cup carrot sticks 2 Tbsp hummus Green Tea			
6	French Toast Full glass of milk. 2 almonds and 2 walnuts	1 large orange 2 graham crackers Green Tea	Honey Lemon Chicken and Brown Rice Pilaf	Any fruit	1-2 bowls of fruit custard.
7	Everything in it burrito and ½ cup canned pineapple chunks	2 whole grain Cookies A tall glass of juice	Bean and Pasta Soup	Any fruit	Cream of Mushroom and Garlic Bread

8	Mediterranean Grain Salad.	Green tea Sprout salad	Red Lentil Soup and Roasted Potato Chops with garlic.	Any fruit	Tofu Stir Fried
9	Blueberry pancakes and a tall glass of cold mocha latte.	Green tea Carrot Sticks with Dip: ½ cup carrot sticks 2 Tbsp hummus	Green Sauce Spaghetti.	Any fruit	Dry chickpea salad.
10	Roasted Vegetables and Feta Sandwiches	Green tea1 large orange	Oven sweet potato fries with mint and coriander	Any fruit	Vegetable and soybean Thukpa

		2 graham crackers	sauce.		
11	Banana Berry Smoothie. Omelette.	Green tea Sprout salad	Classic mac and cheese	Any fruit	Chicken and corn soup.
12	Vegetable and potato vermicelli.	Green tea Carrot Sticks with Dip: ½ cup carrot sticks 2 Tbsp hummus	Tortilla and Black Bean Pie.	Any fruit	Tofu Stir Fried
13	Raisin Oatmeal	Green tea1	Pasta with Parsley-	Any	Egg Sandwich

		large orange 2 graham crackers	Walnut Pesto.	fruit	and Chocolate Mousse.
14	Open-faced Egg and Tomato on an English Muffin	Green tea Sprout salad	Manchurian and Noodles.	Any fruit	Honey Mustard Pork Chops (it's a Sunday)
15	Pumpkin Pancakes and Apple juice.	Green tea Carrot Sticks with Dip: ½ cup carrot sticks 2 Tbsp hummus	Easy Red Beans and Rice	Any fruit	Veggie rice with hot and sour soup.

16	Banana Walnut Oatmeal 1 hard-boiled egg Beverage: 1 cup orange juice	Green tea1 large orange 2 graham crackers	Muffin Meatloaf and Mashed potatoes	Any fruit	Cottage Cheese in onion tomato gravy.
17	Oatmeal and milk with an apple and nuts	Green tea Sprout salad	bread of choice browned in garlic sauce and oil and served with stir fried garlic vegetables.	Any fruit	carrot and tomato soup.
18	French Toast with a cup of	Green tea Carrot	Soybean biryani	Any fruit	Yogurt with tomato

		coffee	Sticks with Dip: ½ cup carrot sticks 2 Tbsp hummus				onion and chilli and oven baked sweet potato
19		Mango Smoothie with nuts and dry cake (from nearby bakery)	Green tea	Lettuce (1 cup) and mushroom spaghetti	Any fruit		Dumplings in clear soup- Thentuk
20		Mix Fruit Bowl and glass of milk	Green tea Sprout salad	Manchurian and Noodles.	Any fruit		Tofu Stir Fried
21		Half fried eggs and Ice Tea	Green tea	Caramelized onion and	Any fruit		Cream of Chicken

		Carrot Sticks with Dip: ½ cup carrot sticks 2 Tbsp hummus	potatoes on white flatbread.		
22	Tofu Salad and green smoothie	Green tea1 large orange 2 graham crackers	Easy Red Beans and Rice	Any fruit	1-2 bowls of fruit custard.
23	Potato Patty in yogurt and coriander mint sauce.	Green tea Sprout	A simple lemon and citrus salad with	Any fruit	Veggie rice with vegetable soup.

		salad	mushroom soup and choice of bread		
24	Sausage Omelet	Green tea Carrot Sticks with Dip: ½ cup carrot sticks 2 Tbsp hummus	Green Salad with Salmon 6 whole-grain crackers Beverage: 1 cup low-fat milk	Any fruit	Banana Bread 1 cup low-fat milk
25	Cereal with Fruit 1 hard-cooked egg Beverage: Water, coffee, tea	Green tea Sprout salad1 large orange 2	Quick Tuna Casserole	Any fruit	One Pan Spaghetti

		graham crackers			
26	Banana Buttermilk Pancakes with butter and maple syrup.	Green tea Carrot Sticks with Dip: ½ cup carrot sticks 2 Tbsp hummus	White Sauce Pasta	Any fruit	Vegetable Stew with poached eggs
27	Muesli or any cereal of choice with milk, a small salad, and nuts.	Green tea1 large orange 2 graham crackers	Soybean biryani	Any fruit	Tomato and olive penne

28	Egg Roll	Sprout salad	Afghani Chicken and flatbread	Any fruit	pasta salad.

MONTH 2:

days	8:00 am breakfast	11:30 am	2:00 pm	AFTER GYM	8:00 pm
1	2 eggs omelette. Full glass of milk. 2 almonds and 2 walnuts	Sprout Salad Green Tea	Dry chickpea salad; boiled cumin and garlic potatoes (1 small potato)	Any fruit	Small salad, egg curry.
2	Chicken Sandwich (No mayo or fatty dressings, use	Carrot Sticks with Dip: ½	Tuna-Cucumber Wrap 5 cucumber	Any fruit	Vegetable soupy oats

	as many vegetables as you can) Orange Juice.	cup carrot sticks 2 Tbsp hummus Green Tea	sticks ¼ cup low-fat vanilla yogurt		
3	1 Blueberry pancake and a small glass of cold mocha latte.	1 large orange 2 graham crackers Green Tea	Yogurt cooked chicken breast.	Any fruit	One Pan Spaghetti (includes turkey and tomato sauce)
4	Muesli or any cereal of choice with milk, a small salad.	Sprout salad Green Tea	Cottage Cheese in onion tomato gravy.	Any fruit	Vegetable and soybean Thukpa
5	Vegetable Sandwich plus a glass of	Carrot Sticks with	Small salad, egg curry, bread 2	Any fruit	Soupy Vegetable

	buttermilk	Dip: ½ cup carrot sticks 2 Tbsp hummus Green Tea	pieces.		Oats
6	French Toast Full glass of milk. 2 almonds and 2 walnuts	1 large orange Green Tea	Honey Lemon Chicken and 1 bread.	Any fruit	1-2 bowls of fruit custard.
7	Everything in it burrito ½ cup canned pineapple chunks	2 whole grain Cookies A tall glass of juice	Bean and Pasta Soup	Any fruit	Cream of Mushroom and Garlic Bread
8	Mediterranean	Green	Red Lentil Soup and	Any	Tofu Stir

	Grain Salad.	tea Sprout salad	Roasted Potato Chops with garlic.	fruit	Fried
9	1 Blueberry pancake and a small glass of cold mocha latte.	Green tea Carrot Sticks with Dip: ½ cup carrot sticks 2 Tbsp hummus	Green Sauce Spaghetti.	Any fruit	Dry chickpea salad.
10	Roasted Vegetables and Feta Sandwiches	Green tea1 large orange 2 graham	White Bean & Herb Hummus with Crudites	Any fruit	Vegetable and soybean Thukpa

		crackers			
11	Banana Berry Smoothie. Omelette.	Green tea Sprout salad	BBQ Turkey Burgers	Any fruit	Chicken and corn soup.
12	Vegetable and potato vermicelli.	Green tea Carrot Sticks with Dip: ½ cup carrot sticks 2 Tbsp hummus	Tortilla and Black Bean Pie.	Any fruit	Tofu Stir Fried
13	Raisin Oatmeal	Green tea1 large	Pasta with Parsley-Walnut	Any fruit	Egg Sandwich and Chocolate

		orange	Pesto.		Mousse.
		2 graham crackers			
14	Open-faced Egg and Tomato on an English Muffin	Green tea Sprout salad	Manchurian and Noodles.	Any fruit	Honey Mustard Pork Chops (it's a Sunday)
15	Pumpkin Pancakes and Apple juice.	Green tea Carrot Sticks with Dip: ½ cup carrot sticks 2 Tbsp hummus	Easy Red Beans and Rice	Any fruit	Veggie rice with hot and sour soup.

16	Banana Walnut Oatmeal 1 hard-boiled egg Beverage: 1 cup orange juice	Green tea1 large orange 2 graham crackers	Middle Eastern Rice Salad	Any fruit	Cottage Cheese in onion tomato gravy.
17	Breakfast Barley with Banana & Sunflower Seeds	Green tea Sprout salad	bread of choice browned in garlic sauce and oil and served with stir fried garlic vegetables.	Any fruit	carrot and tomato soup.
18	French Toast with a cup of	Green tea Carrot	Curried Egg Salad Sandwich	Any fruit	Yogurt with tomato

		coffee	Sticks with Dip: ½ cup carrot sticks 2 Tbsp hummus			onion and chilli and oven baked sweet potato
19	Salmon Noodle Bowl	Green tea1 large orange 2 graham crackers	Lettuce (1 cup) and mushroom spaghetti	Any fruit	Dumplings in clear soup- Thentuk	
20	Mix Fruit Bowl and glass of milk	Green tea Sprout salad	Manchurian and Noodles.	Any fruit	Tofu Stir Fried	

21	Half fried eggs and Ice Tea	Green tea Carrot Sticks with Dip: ½ cup carrot sticks 2 Tbsp hummus	Caramelized onion and potatoes on white flatbread.	Any fruit	Cream of Chicken
22	Tofu Salad and green smoothie	Green tea1 large orange 2 graham crackers	Easy Red Beans and Rice	Any fruit	1-2 bowls of fruit custard.

| 23 | Potato Patty in yogurt and coriander mint sauce. | Green tea

Sprout salad | A simple lemon and citrus salad with mushroom soup and choice of bread | Any fruit | Veggie rice with vegetable soup. |
| 24 | Sausage Omelet | Green tea

Carrot Sticks with

Dip: ½ cup carrot sticks 2 Tbsp hummus | Green Salad with Salmon

6 whole-grain crackers

Beverage: 1 cup low-fat milk | Any fruit | Banana Bread

1 cup low-fat milk |
| 25 | Cereal with Fruit

1 hard-cooked | Green tea1 large | Quick Tuna Casserole | Any fruit | One Pan Spaghetti |

	egg Beverage: Water, coffee, tea	orange 2 graham crackers			
26	Banana Buttermilk Pancakes with butter and maple syrup.	Green tea Sprout salad	White Sauce Pasta	Any fruit	Vegetable Stew with poached eggs
27	Muesli or any cereal of choice with milk, a small salad, and nuts.	Green tea Carrot Sticks with Dip: ½ cup carrot sticks 2 Tbsp hummus	Pan-Grilled Salmon with Pineapple Salsa	Any fruit	Tomato and olive penne

28	Egg Roll	Green tea 1 large orange 2 graham crackers	Afghani Chicken and flatbread	Any fruit	pasta salad.

4.   BUSY? WE'VE GOT YOUR BACK!

It's the 21st century and every darn good human being on earth is running; running to make a livelihood, to better the state of this planet, its economy and what not. In such a haphazard lifestyle, with so many deadlines to meet and meetings to follow, it's pretty easy to forget to take care of oneself and of one's health. Late night drinks, unprepared dining outs, early mornings mess and so on and so forth.

But we greatly care about the lives of our busy readers and would love to give some healthy eating tips to keep their metabolic gears grinding while simultaneously maintaining their timid office timings.

-Breakfast is indispensable. Never rely on caffeine!

As is said, a couple of chapters ago, breakfast is the first and the foremost meal of the day to kick-start your body-automobile. You wake up every morning and need energy and missing out on breakfast may be the most excruciating thing you may be doing to your health. Oatmeal and whole grain bread are just the jam. Add some fruits to make them the perfect meal. Lay off a high carb or a high sugar breakfast, though. That just jumbles up the blood sugar. Also, caffeine feels like a necessity sometimes but believe us, you need to curfew that dark-tongue-grabbing beverage right now. Coffee dehydrates the body excessively and overloads the liver. A tasty alternative is an herbal tea. Soothing for the throat and healthy for the system!

-Always, always keep yourself hydrated!

Most people do not know, or maybe pretty much indifferent to it, but hydration is one of the most crucial states of your whole digestive cycle. Water, as simple and tasteless it may be, holds an account to two-thirds of your body. Always keep a water bottle close to you and keep yourselves hydrated. When the body is in a state of dehydration, it confuses with a feeling of hunger. Avoid cold water and drink normal temperature water as cold water causes gastrointestinal contractions and slows the digestion down. Roughly eight glasses of water will keep your metabolism up, and your appetite down, allowing you to concentrate more on your work and less on your hunger.

-Limit your alcohol intake to a minimum.

Alcohol is one clumsy dehydrator. It lowers the inhibitions and heavily increases the appetite (talk about those munchies...) and everything else since we are talking of the triggered munchies. Nutritionists always advise drinking a glass of water for each alcoholic beverage you consume. An average male should keep his daily drinking quota to two drinks while an average female, one. Non-alcoholic drinks, on the other hand, are usually suggested with a happy heart by every food expert. Light beer, or sparkling water, or just a glass of concentrated lemonade are all healthy alternatives to alcohol. If you're embarrassed about what your colleagues might think, just ask for your drink in a tumbler.

-Say no to overeating.

This is by far the most common problem working people face. Overeating. The mid-day meals are nowhere to be found and their metabolism stops to the point where they're so hungry that they'll eat a wooden door. This sudden shoving of food causes overeating. It's advised that one should eat until he/she is sufficiently sufficed. Eat up till you're 70 percent full and no more. If after a few minutes, you're still hungry, then eat a little more. When you overeat, you not only gain weight sufficiently but you slow down your digestion process which may lead to problems like diabetes.

-Always keep snacks with you and eat fruits/vegetables more.

Since you'll be out for more than a while, always keep a fruit piece or a nut bar or some healthy protein bar in your bag. Having small meals occasionally throughout the day keeps the metabolism of the body intact and also reduces the possibility of overeating by keeping the appetite in check.

Also, fruits and vegetables are the colorful pool of nutrients you can fill yourselves with. 2-3 fruit servings and 5-7 vegetable servings are decently healthy. Spinach, kale, and other greens are surely advised as they pack the most nutrients.

-Stick to whole foods.

Fresh meat, fish, grains, seeds, nuts, vegetables, and fruits are what our previous generations relied on. Good health is what you get by consuming whole foods. If you wanna bring something to snack upon during your office, bring a fruit, veggies or a nut bar. Best snack ever!

-Avoid packaged, refined foods.

Packaged foods are always packed with salts, sugars, stabilizers, preservatives and flavored ingredients of all kinds. They also contain artificial colors which have an unnoticeable but adverse effect on your health. A good rule of thumb is if you find even one name in the list of ingredients difficult to pronounce, skip the food. Also, choose your food item by the number of ingredients in it. The fewer the better.

So these are pretty much them. A brief list of eating habits that all you fast-lane-workers may comfortably slide in your lifestyle to keep up with a good health without compromising your work life.

5.   OVERWEIGHT? A THING OF THE PAST.

Overweight people are probably the most frustrated people on earth. They are frustrated because of their slow metabolisms, their over the top love for food and various other reasons which we are not going deep into because we want to talk about the ways we can change the situation. But you do not need to be. The problem might be that you have never put that extra effort which was required but yeah! The metabolism thingy just sucks!! There are ways you can boost up your metabolism, though. Read along!

Honestly, you can lose 10-15 pounds in 2 months if you do nothing else and simply follow the meal plan above. Otherwise here are a few things you can do to shift into a healthier lifestyle!

- Cut down seriously on your carb consumption!
- Carb consumption should be about 15-25% of the total food consumption in a day!
- Quit these things: Soda, binge eating (explained later in the book), sugary treats and M&Ms.
- Eat the carbohydrate you need before and after workout
- Drink 3-4 cups of green tea during the day. Add lemon to enhance the flavour and effects.
- Try drinking black coffee before working out, would increase stamina and make you burn more calories!

We want to keep this section short because a lot of books have just catered to the problems of overweight people and left other issues untouched, so that is why we would be moving on to rarely talked about issues in respect to overweight people.

6. SUPER SKINNY? JUST READ ALONG...

Well, you're too thin and you hate that? No worries. That doesn't stop you from eating healthy. Although whenever the topic of skinny people eating healthy comes in motion, the thought comes to the mind that will it not cause weight loss? Mostly healthy eating naturally causes weight loss, but healthy eating is not a term that has limited instructions, it has varied implications for various kinds of people. So, in a way it causes weight loss but also allows the body to work in a healthier atmosphere which is necessary for a longer life with lesser diseases. So keeping the latter in mind the weight loss aspect can be tackled. How do we do this? There are two things that people need to keep in mind even while being skinny! You might look skinny but there are chances that your body has some toxic or bad layers of fat. These are the layers you don't wanna keep in your body even when you know you will lose some amounts of fat which you don't want to. This is the reason many people don't healthy eat and actually many 'skinny' people!

So in our case here, healthy eating first will detoxify your body by losing the bad fat and then will go on strengthening your body. The time when the body strengthens is when you will regain all the fat stores your body previously had. Well, this was too direct to say! Because till yet we have not gone down to the cause of the problem, the problem of you being so skinny that people start calling you 'the kid with malnutrition'! So our biggest problem when we talk about the causes of being skinny is the fire struck metabolism you have! Is that a good thing or a bad thing? Many people have asked us. Our answer: Good metabolism is an awesome thing. Yes, we believe that a higher than average metabolism never harms someone because ultimately people can eat more to compensate the activity done by their systems.

Why is a higher metabolism a good thing? This is because you would not have to worry about your body unable to process carbs and other heavy complex materials that we eat around. The very reason that some people have always been fat is the presence of a slow metabolic system which makes fat burn much slowly. Their bodies have adapted to low energy conditions and also adapted to the layers of the fat present while people with fiery metabolisms have to keep their instant energy drinks with themselves always because their bodies have not adapted to low energy conditions and also do not have any stored fat. So that is the reason skinny people are always up for some high fructose corn syrup filled soda, which actually is very harmful whenever you drink something with it.

Coming to the point then, what exactly do you do to eat healthily?

The following points have the practical tips which can really bring a change in how your body looks and lives in the longer run.

• So we made this long talk about metabolism, we gather that we will have to tackle metabolism in our own way, that we don't have to allow the metabolism to burn all the fat stores in our bodies which also are emergency fat stores. For that, the number one thing you have to keep in mind is the knowledge of how metabolism exactly works. So it targets the macronutrients which are easy to break, so the number one nutrient here is the 'Carbohydrate'. Carbs are broken down first and converted into energy fastest. So it goes like this: the body first converts carbs, then it converts proteins and finally fats. In order to save your muscles which get depleted easily than the fat on your body, you need to keep yourself all fuelled up! For that, you need to take in a lot of carbs as they are the ones which provide instant energy. Our next point explains how to take carbs properly.

• There are many types of carbohydrates one can consume. There are simpler carbs and complex carbs. The simple ones are sugar and other mono or disaccharides technically while the complex ones are fibres and starches, etc. Simpler ones get digested easily and provide energy instantly. A healthy diet should be a proper mixture of both the things. While you should consume nuts as carbohydrates, it is important that you do not consume many, because they are mostly fats but have some complex carbohydrate in them. So if you consume 4-5 pieces in the morning, do not consume then during the rest of the day.

- What simple carbs you must consume? Sugar is what will make your energy levels alleviate instantly. Consuming the right kinds of sugars is really important! Earlier in this paragraph, we talked about high fructose corn syrups! They are the enemies. The real enemies! When you consume soda, your body takes a lot of high fructose corn syrup. This sugar has the ability to cause high blood pressure, type-2 diabetes, glucose intolerance if done in the long term. So reduce that intake. So consume fruits, fruit juices, tea or coffee in a moderate amount is never harmful.

- What complex carbs you must consume? Pasta, Bread or anything starchy. Cake maybe? So yes these products provide energy and unlike simple carbohydrates, these are not just empty calories, they also contain some protein, some fats, and also some vitamins and minerals. Also, make sure the flour used to make these things is whole, not refined. When you will quit refined flour you will naturally shift to a healthier lifestyle as the whole grains contain a lot of minerals and vitamins with them.

- How to consume fats and proteins? Well consume a lot of protein, your metabolism is so high that it does not allow your muscle to stay and thus making you look even thinner. Have a lot of eggs, and do not worry about the yolk, the yolk has a lot of B vitamins. Consume chicken, fish, and meat products as they will help you build the muscle that sustains.

About fat, go for only healthier options. Have a lot of omega-3s and omega-6s because our body does not really produce them and that is why they come in the category of essential fatty acids. Consume nuts and olive oil in your salads. So all in all the some of the healthy options for you to consume are avocados, butter (the real one), coconut oil, etc. You're skinny and you can have anything so increase your capacity to eat and binge on salads, juices, and normal food.

7. EMOTIONAL BINGE EATING? NO NEED TO WORRY ABOUT!

Oh, this is our favourite part of the book. Binge eaters are people full of love. And do not worry because the tips in this section of the book are really going to help you get out of this habit of binge eating. Binge eating is due to a lot of causes, because of being angry, or sometimes being sad or depressed or elated and extremely happy. One thing that is common in all the above is emotions. So basically what we are targeting here is 'emotional binge eating' because that one is the hardest to get under control because hey you cannot get your thoughts under control, can you? So we need to get this mental psychological activity related with emotional extremes under control. It is like our brain should get another signal whenever it comes under emotional crisis, a signal which does not direct towards eating food. For that you need to follow this strategy:

- Dieting is not the option. Why do we emphasise on this so much? Because most people who are patients of binge eating disorders have stated that they were trying to diet mostly and when the diets did not work out (because we all know, dieting is crazy, hard, unreal, and unhealthy) they spiralled into eating more and more of what they were eating before. The emotions involved here were of disappointment and anger. So now you know what not to do, just do not go for crazy dieting.

- Add into your binge eating routine only instead of fussing over what to not eat because the latter only creates more problems. Add healthy things to your food. Instead of keeping bourbons at your place, start keeping juices and instead of chocolates and ice-creams eat salads and vegetable casseroles. It will be like you are preparing to binge eat. How can this help? Well you are in a crisis and you decide to eat this because that is all you have around you at that time, but then after you feel better emotionally you no longer have the post eating guilt which always engulfs you. You will less often fall prey to the vicious circle of eating if you stick to this experimental idea.

- We, as author of this book do not really promote cheat days! See cheat days are for people who are naturally very controlled who do not even 'cheat' like it's a cheat day. For binge eaters, cheat days can be triggering points in a schedule where they have been trying hard to fight binge eating.

- IGNORE THE MINOR SETBACKS: Well we believe that people can have perfect days, perfect weeks but not a perfect life when perfect equals eating according to book. So there will be days when you will be busy way too much to focus on your food or workout which is okay, you don't have to be disheartened by that and carry on the next day. There might even be a week where you were neither able to diet properly and you probably were travelling and hence could not either workout, so what do you do? Do you become sad and angry that nothing is working out and you are never able to do it? You just have to resume the next day. We do not use the word 'start over' because you never stopped anything, life came in between and you paused. So you do not 'start over' after pausing, you just 'resume' without being overwhelmed.

- Since binge eating is an emotional problem and therefore the solution also should be somewhere in the emotions. For a longer riddance of this issue, you need to find support in something other than food. Oh and we totally do not mean alcohol. We mean people. Find support in positive human beings who motivate you towards your causes who understand that binge eating is a problem and not shun for what you are. So do not go for people who tell you 'Oh binge eating! It is not even a problem, it is you who are hungry and cannot control it'. We have seen so many people like this we cannot even think the world actually exists with people who understand us. Well do not let this be the cause of your sadness and just be positive from the inside and try finding out people you connect with, it could even be strangers, it always is strangers.

- In this diet book about healthy living, you would have rarely seen us as prescribing exact foods and diet plans. Instead, our major focus remains on deciphering problems and understanding the root causes because this book is mostly about fitting in a healthy lifestyle for a longer life. And anything which needs to be adopted for the longer run has to be tackled deeply which requires coming to a comfortable and non-extreme solution. That is why we are telling you to adopt the food you will love in future. Understand what you like and what you do not. You know the right kind of foods, like the good fats and that you will benefit by eating more proteins and vegetables and fruits compared to the McDonald's junk.

8. MANAGING ALCOHOL IN THE COOLEST WAY POSSIBLE!

Now since we are here talking about the practical tips on how to turn towards healthy eating for a longer life then we cannot really avoid the fact that alcohol is approximately equal to a beverage in our consumption system. Well, it has been there for years and though we ourselves do not advocate alcohol, we sure advocate realism and optimization. The extremist approach is what you should never go for. Though it is never a bad idea to quit alcohol in life if you think you are the addicting type! So how do you optimize alcohol and why should you not drastically take steps like removing alcohol totally if you have been doing it for a longer time.

There are many ways to optimize alcohol! Here are a few points you should know:

- Just save it for the parties! Well, if you have settled down in your life and have proudly passed your college and bachelor phase of life then we can bet there would be a significant reduction in the number of parties because let's face it; every day at college is a party day! Also when you are a bachelor and are in college, you don't drink in a classy manner you drink, do something crazy and make every night memorable. So, we happily salute the college spirit and proudly move on to the sober and responsible phase of life with reduced parties and controlled drinking. Yeah, that just sounds normal. Well, but if you are not doing this then one thing we suggest - you sit back and analyze. See if you are handling it all well, and that do you really need to be a bit more responsible now, or this excessive drinking might lead to addiction which obviously can cause serious health implications and also family issues in the future. So ease your intake. Make it a deal that you would only drink it in the parties or never ever. You would naturally feel better and will be able to control your alcohol intake anytime you want.

- Well, if you do not want to be such a controlling person over yourself and honestly do not want your friends to call you a jerk every time you do not drink some pints with them, then have more self-control. 'Drink Lightly'. Many people do not even know the distinction between drinking lightly and moderately. For some reason, we have had clients who think 3 to 4 pints of beer is considered light drinking because that is when they start to feel dizzy and buzzed. What actually is the number then? You will be actually pretty shocked when you know what the real limit is! Moderately drinking according to the dietary guidelines for Americans will be one drink for the ladies and two for the gentlemen. So, if you also thought that 3 to 4 pints is the real number then that is probably you have been consuming alcohol for a long time which has given you the tolerance you never needed. It is always good to get buzzed from that second pint or that first peg of the fine scotch. Added benefit saves you some money while allowing you to sip on the finest of drinks. Well and since many studies have shown that drinking alcohol might actually reduce the occurrence of the infamous cardiovascular diseases by 25-40%, it is not that bad to have a drink daily. If you already do so, you may as well do it in good spirit. If that information is hard to believe you should go on Google scholar and read a few research articles on the good benefits. Trust us, they are there.

- Now comes the third category, the ones who are addicted to drinking. Well, you guys have the best chance of improving because there is a lot of space for improving. Chances are your liver is in bad condition and so is the rest of your body because that gland has a huge dependency. What should you do? Nothing that we can suggest but since you are reading this book and you probably thought of changing some habits, then we suggest you simply go to a rehab centre and do as they say. Then it is just a matter of 2-3 months if the determination is firm. Stay Healthy, Stay Fit!

9.   CONCLUSION. PERIOD.

So after all the brilliant information we have talked about in this book, time is to conclude something out of all. So we love our conclusions to be in a manner of a nice schedule.

So, it is a brilliant morning and you have gotten up, have a tall glass of warm water with lemon. It is still the best hack to wake up our systems. Then go for a short run if you do not have time, come home get some bath and have a heavy but healthy breakfast. Pick up anything from the meal plan. Try including a bowl of fruits and milk! Then head where ever you need to, work and have green teas, and then have a moderate lunch. Get home, workout and eat an after workout snack which can be high in calories but the skinny people do not need to worry, they can have a calorie food anytime in a day but like a prescription. Keep the dinner as light as possible with mostly proteins and vegetables!

Sleep at a legit time because if the sleep is compromised, the hunger hormone is released which is widely known by the name of 'leptin' and causes people to eat anything that comes in sight! Bad hormone! You don't want that. And then you repeat the schedule. Happy eating ☺

We sincerely hope you loved the book and that this will impart good vibes to your life.

www.ingramcontent.com/pod-product-compliance
Lightning Source LLC
Chambersburg PA
CBHW060222290526
45789CB00003B/1369